I'm Ready To Learn About

SAFETY

by
Imogene Forte

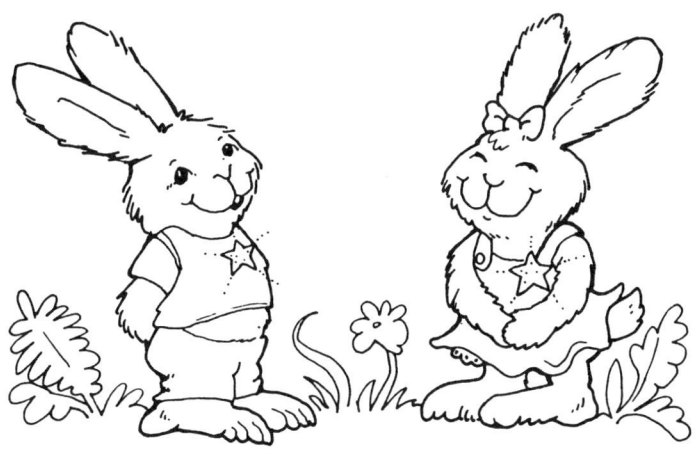

Illustrated by Gayle Seaberg Harvey
Cover illustration by Francis Huffman
Edited by Jennifer Goodman

ISBN 0-86530-120-4

TO PARENTS AND TEACHERS

Why You Need This Book

- The READY TO LEARN SERIES capitalizes on the vitally important "teachable" years from 3-5.
- Basic skills and concepts are introduced to help pave the way to increased self-confidence and life-long learning success.

What Children Will Learn From This Book

- Children will learn basic rules to follow which deal with:
  —personal safety
  —fire safety
  —street and bicycle safety
  —play safety

How To Get The Most From This Book

- Read and interpret the directions for your child.
- Keep the atmosphere light and relaxed.
- Allow the child to work at his or her own pace, free from pressure to perform.
- Praise the child's efforts!

BONUS

See the suggested activities at the back of this book to extend and reinforce the skills and concepts learned.

_____

- -

_____

is ready to learn about

SAFETY

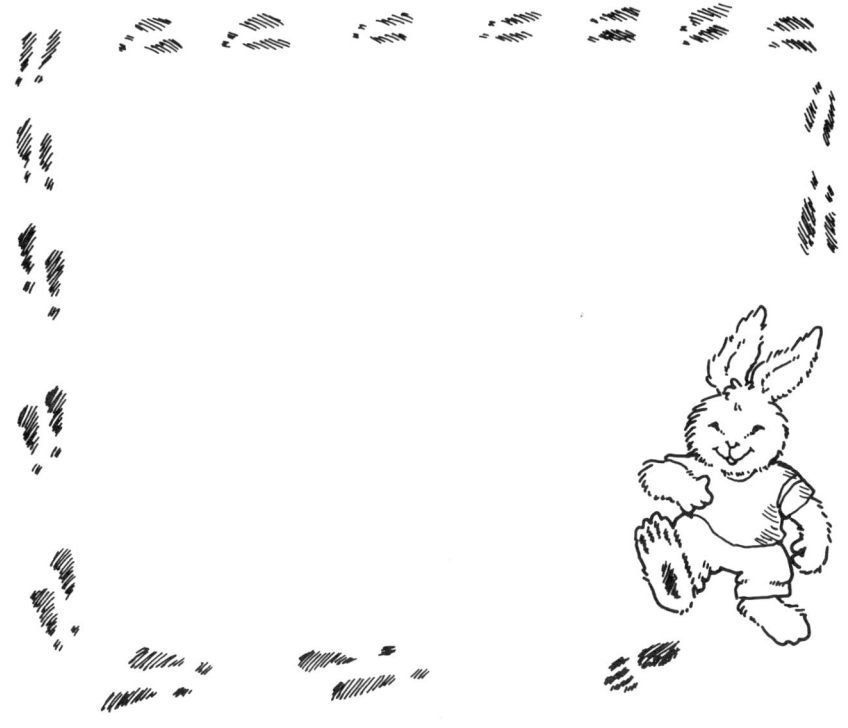

Put your fingerprints here so that the
people who care about you will
always have a record of them.
Use a pad of ink or some thin paint to
make the prints.

It is important to know your:

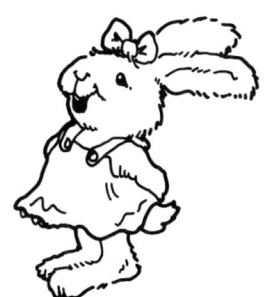

Name:

- -

Address:

- -

- -

Telephone Number:

- -

Understanding personal safety
©1986 by Incentive Publications, Inc., Nashville, TN.

Draw dot-to-dot to find the telephone. Write a number below that you can call in emergencies.

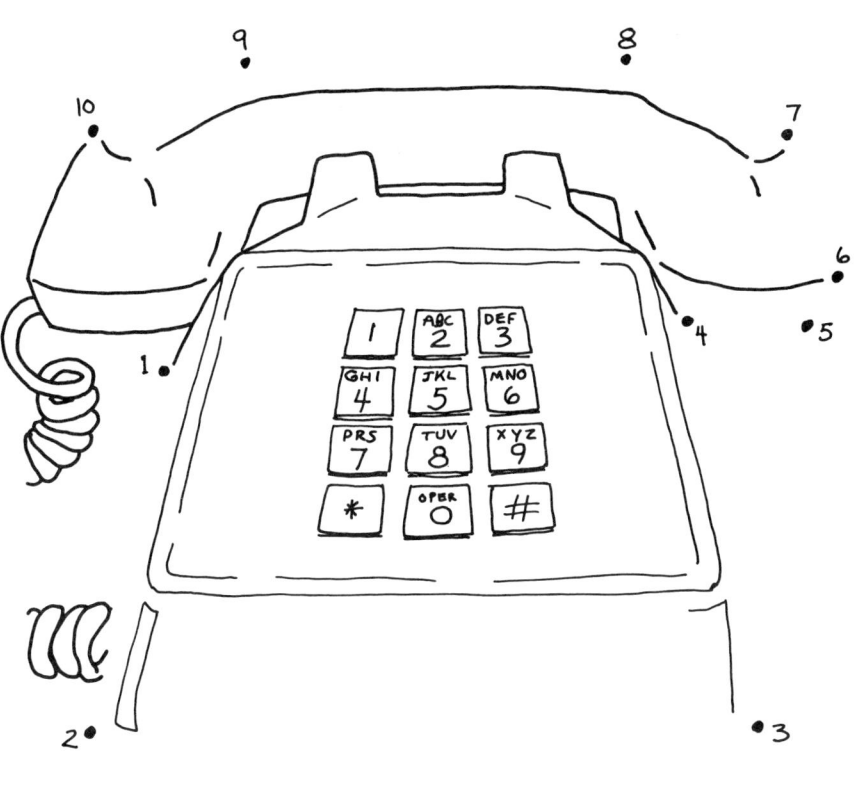

If you cut yourself, stop the bleeding by
pressing your hand on the cut.
Then call for help.
Pretend that you have cut yourself and
do what Tony is doing.
Color the picture.

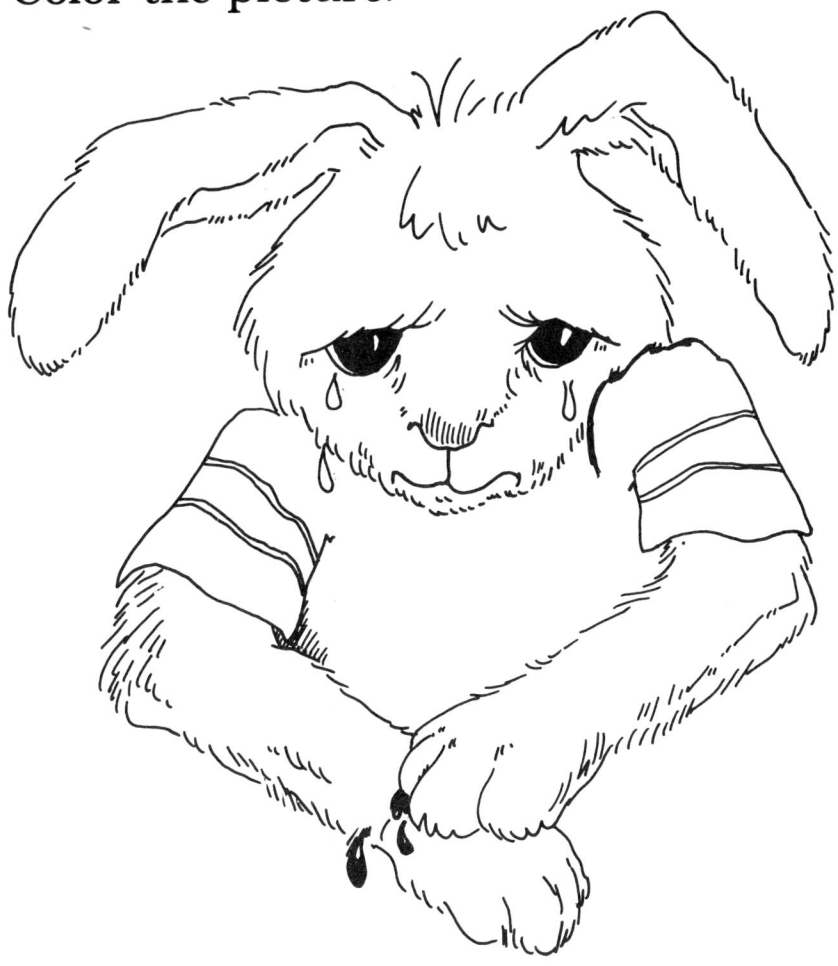

Understanding personal safety
©1986 by Incentive Publications, Inc., Nashville, TN.

Medicine is for sick people.
Never take medicine by yourself.
Help Tonya find her Mom so that she can take her medicine.

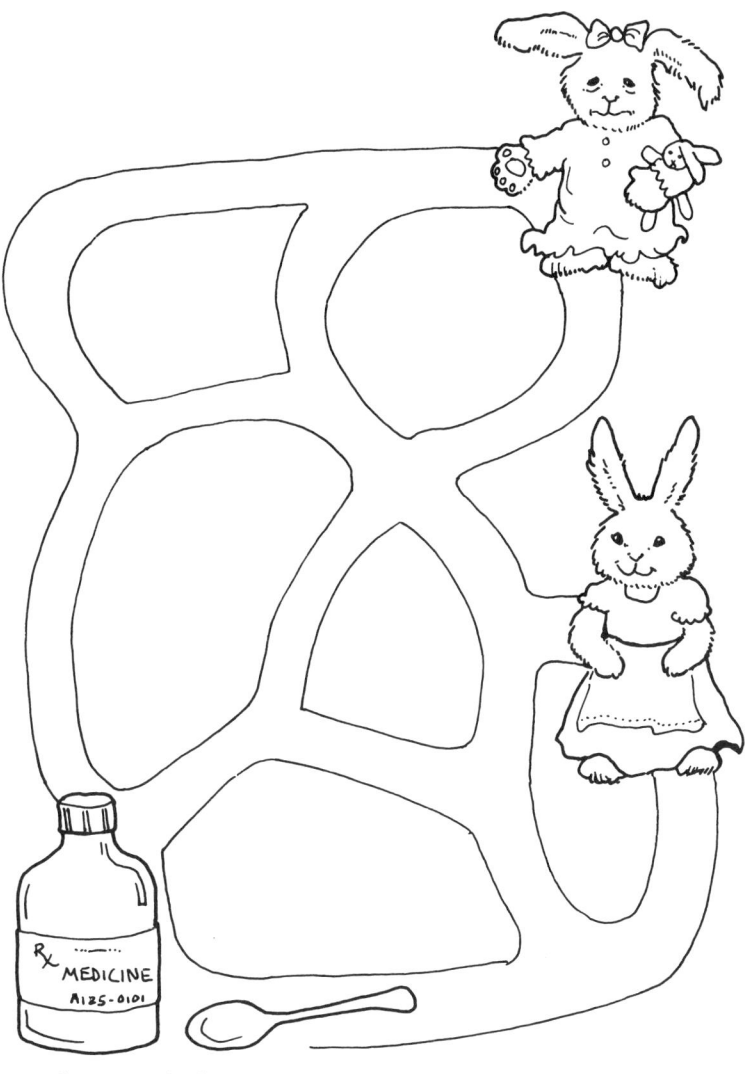

Be careful what you drink!
Always ask permission first.
This symbol means danger.
Mark the dangerous liquids.

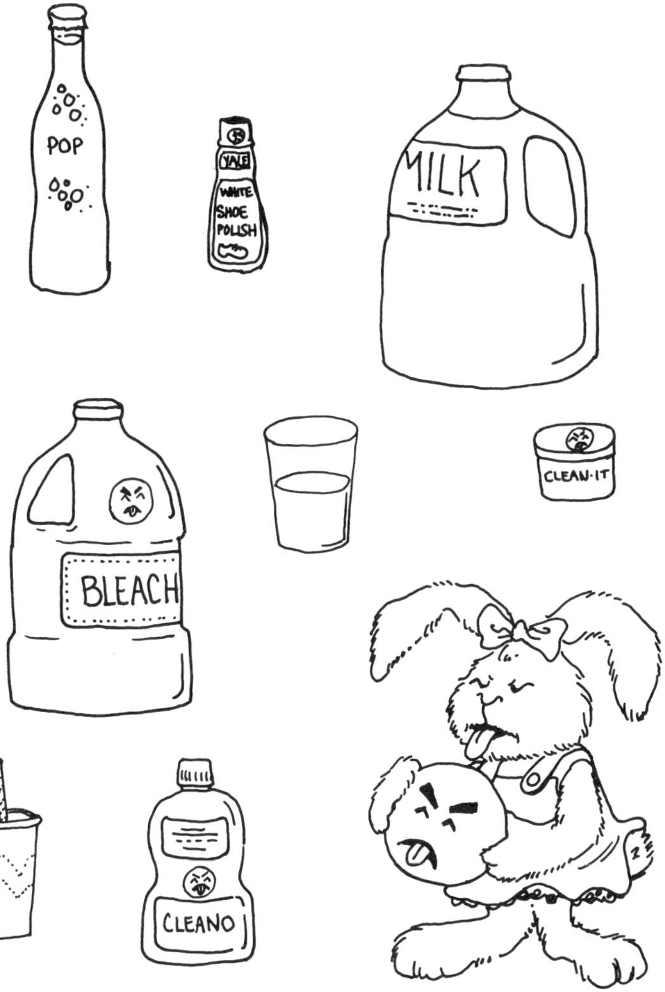

Never touch the top of a hot stove! It might burn you. Cut out these pieces and put them together to make a stove.

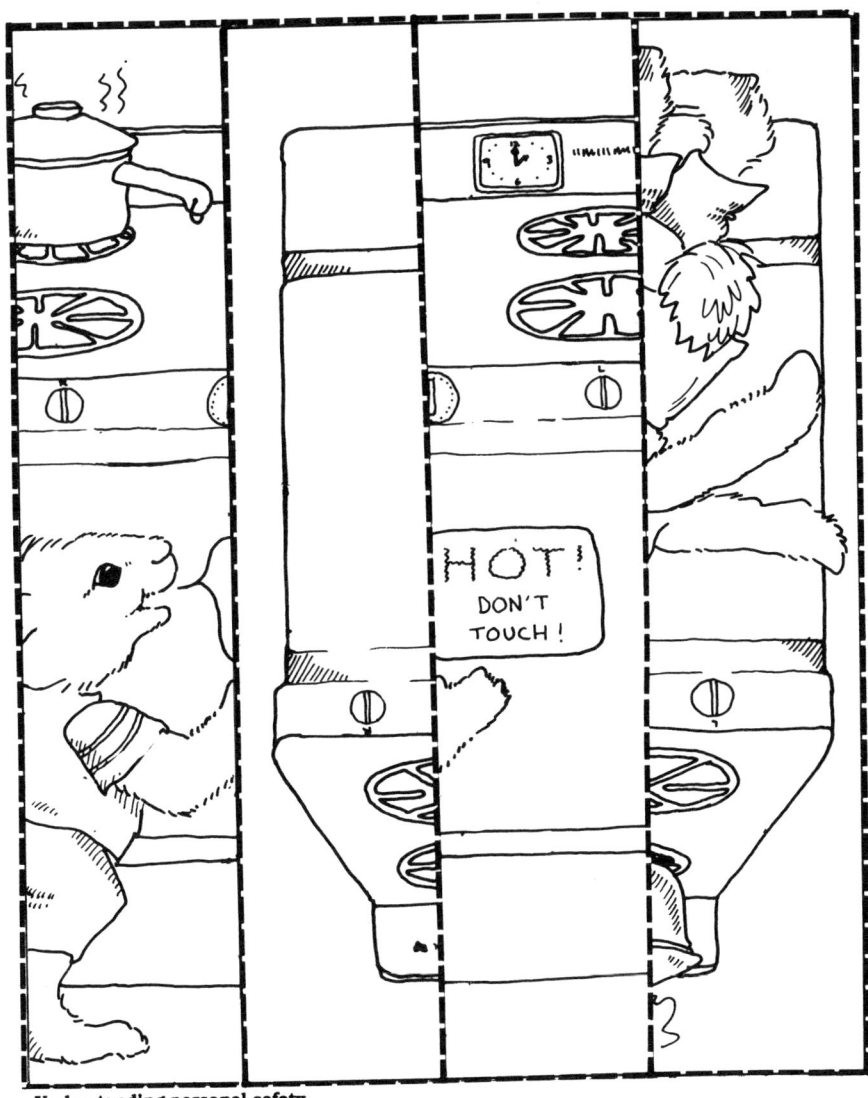

Stay with the adult in charge when you go shopping.
Mark the picture of the boy who is not being careful.

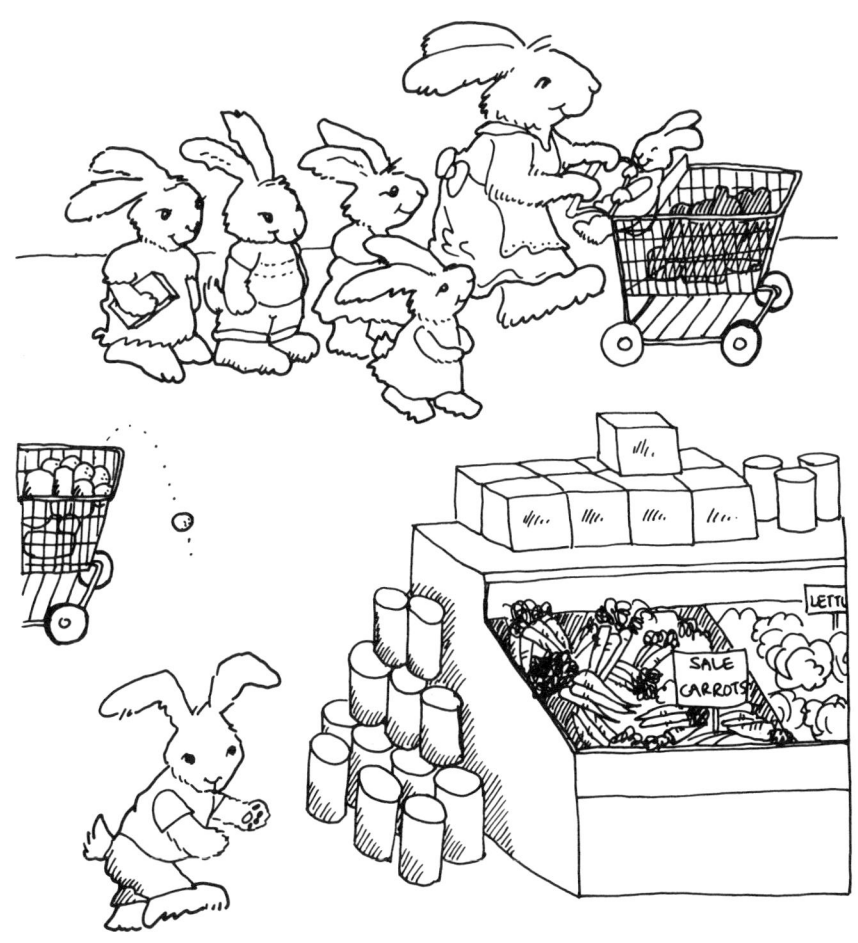

Check the safety rules below that you always follow.

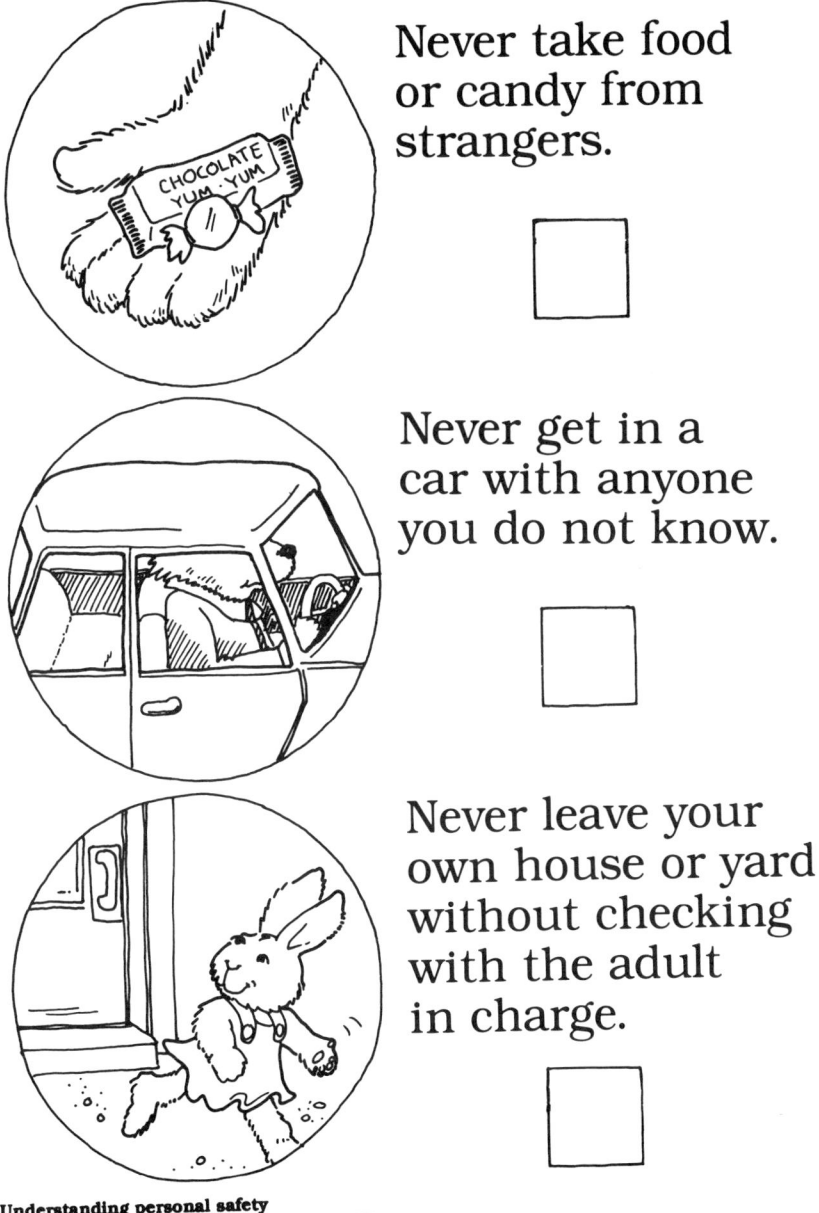

Never take food or candy from strangers.

Never get in a car with anyone you do not know.

Never leave your own house or yard without checking with the adult in charge.

Toys left lying out can cause accidents. Color the toys that should be put away.

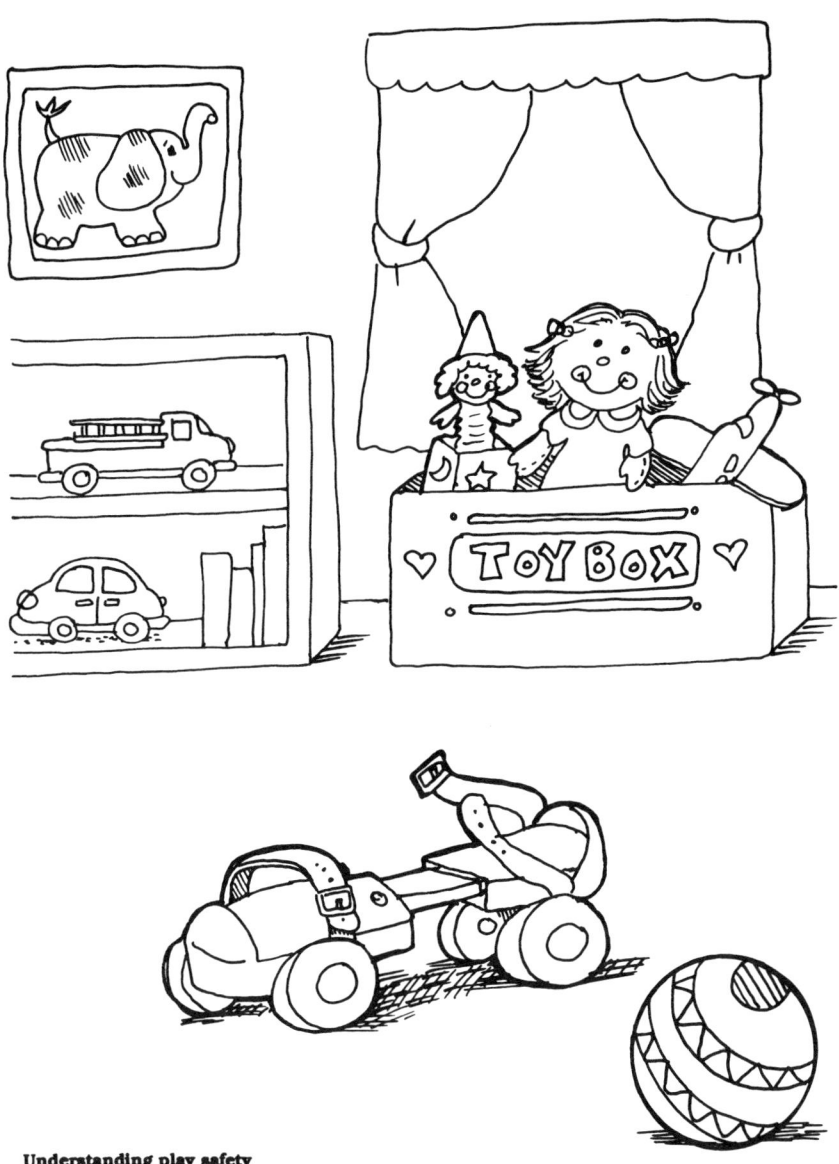

Rusty, broken toys can be harmful. Circle the harmful toys.

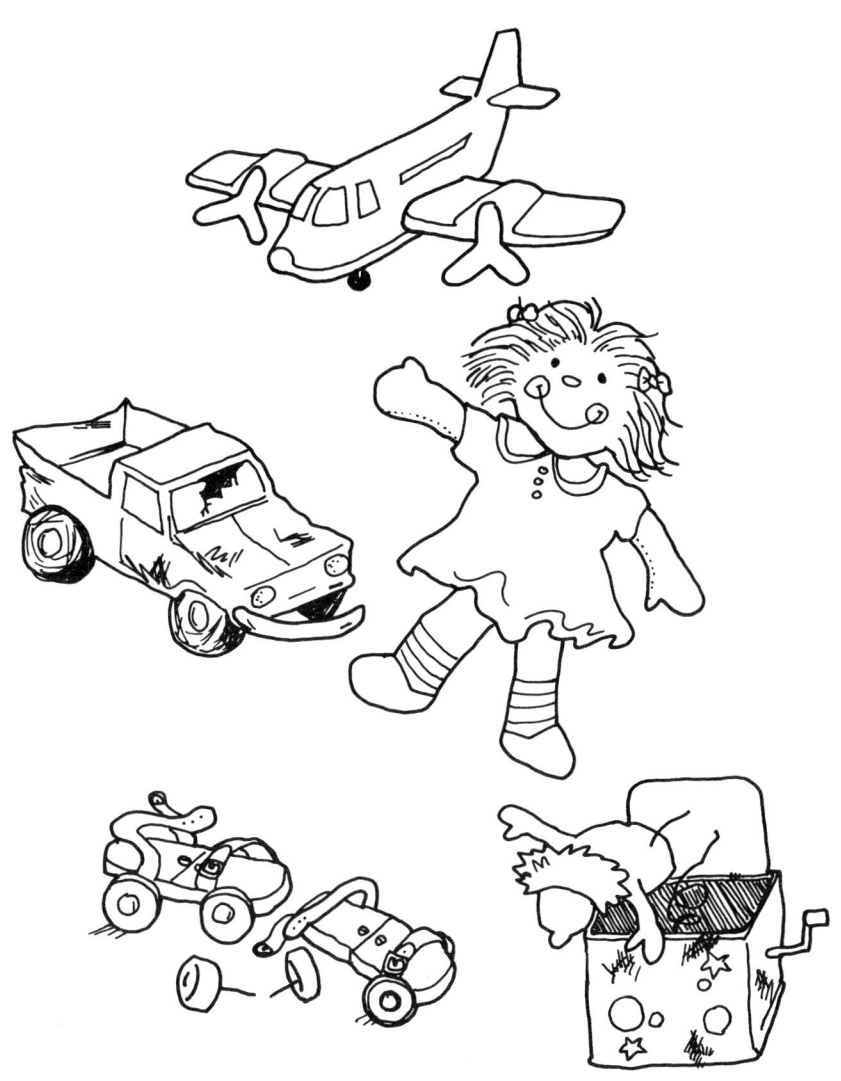

Understanding play safety
©1986 by Incentive Publications, Inc., Nashville, TN.

Don't pet strange animals.
They may not be friendly.
Help Tony find the way home.

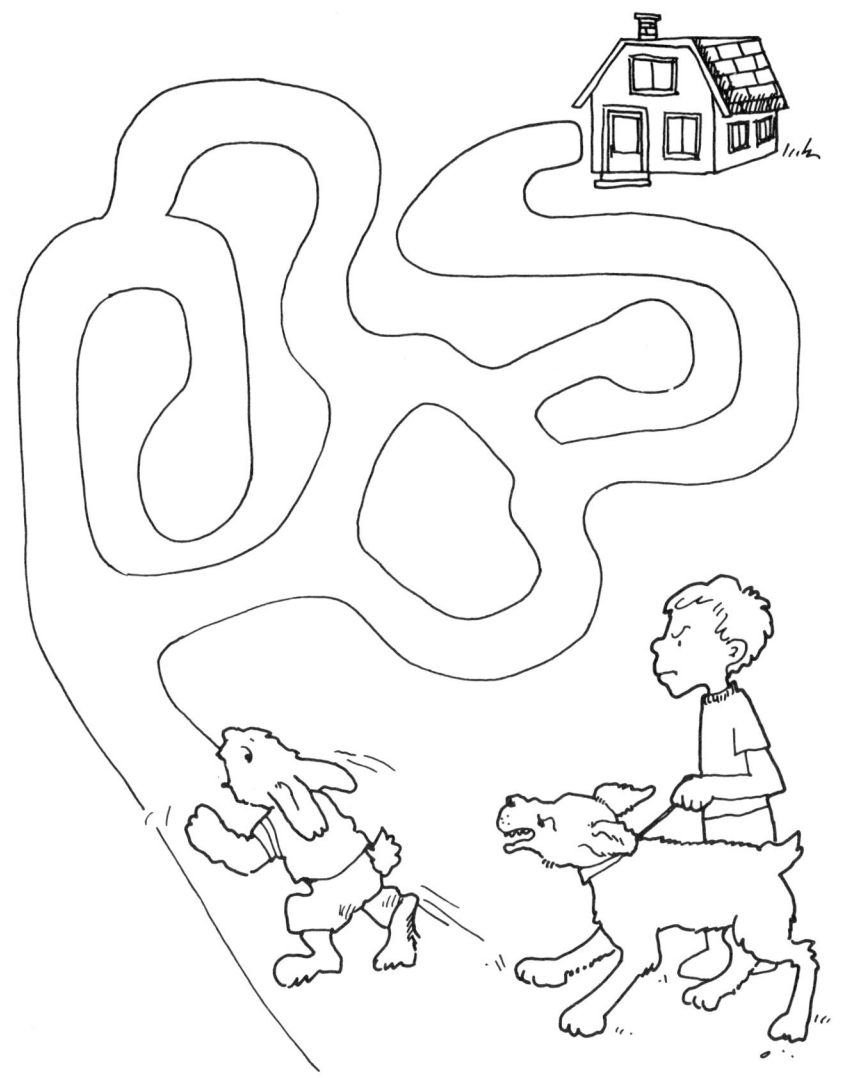

Understanding play safety
©1986 by Incentive Publications. Inc.. Nashville. TN.

Poison ivy looks lovely, but watch out,
you might be allergic to it.
Color the poison ivy green.

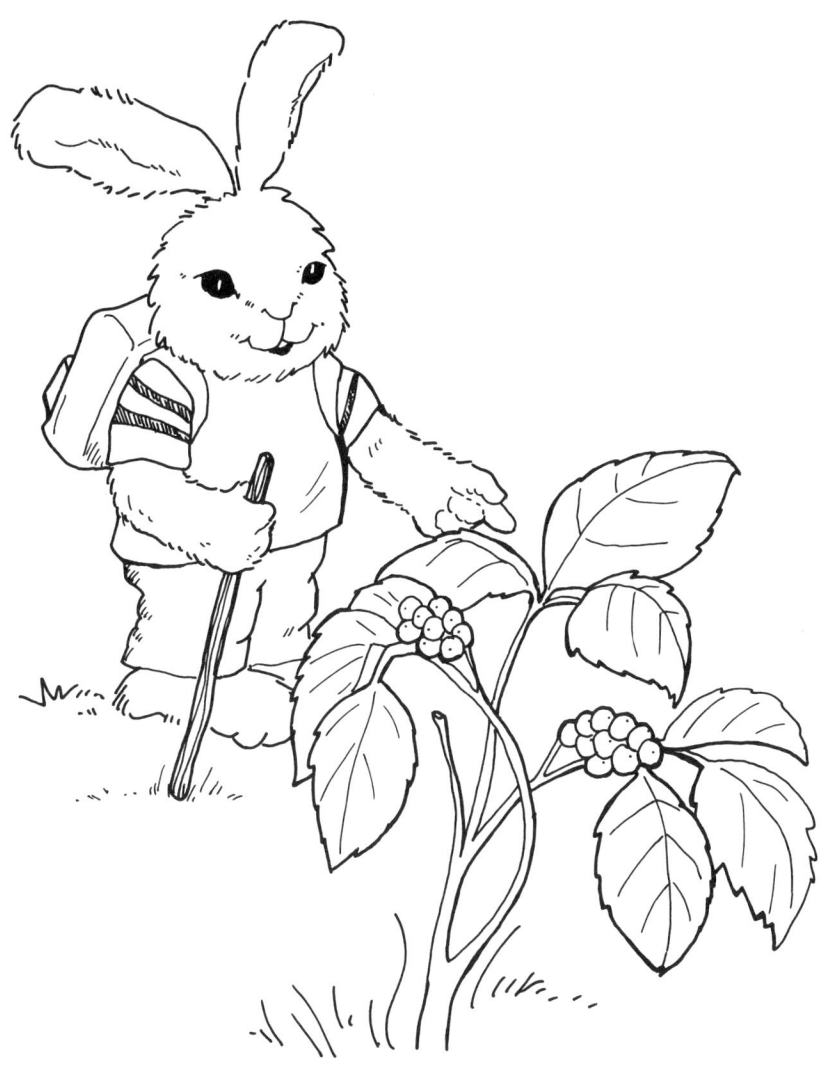

Stay away from electrical sockets.
You might get shocked!
Circle objects which should not go into an electrical socket.

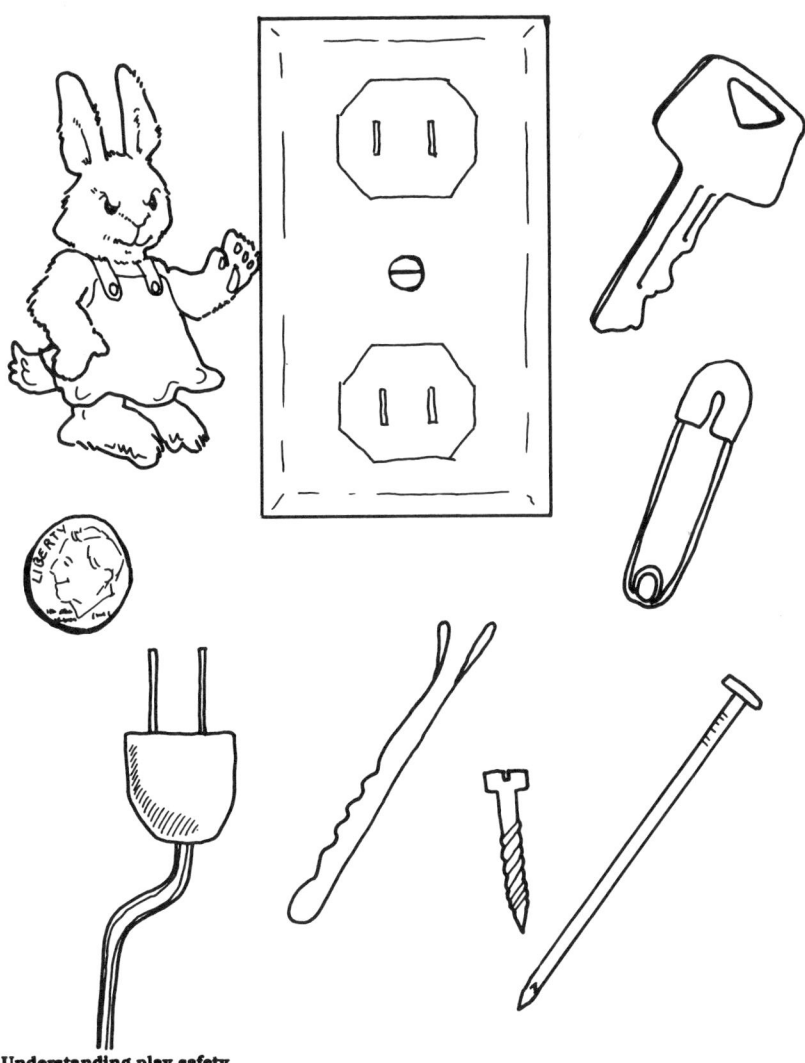

Beware of these!
They might bite or sting.
Mark each with an X to remind you
to stay away from them.

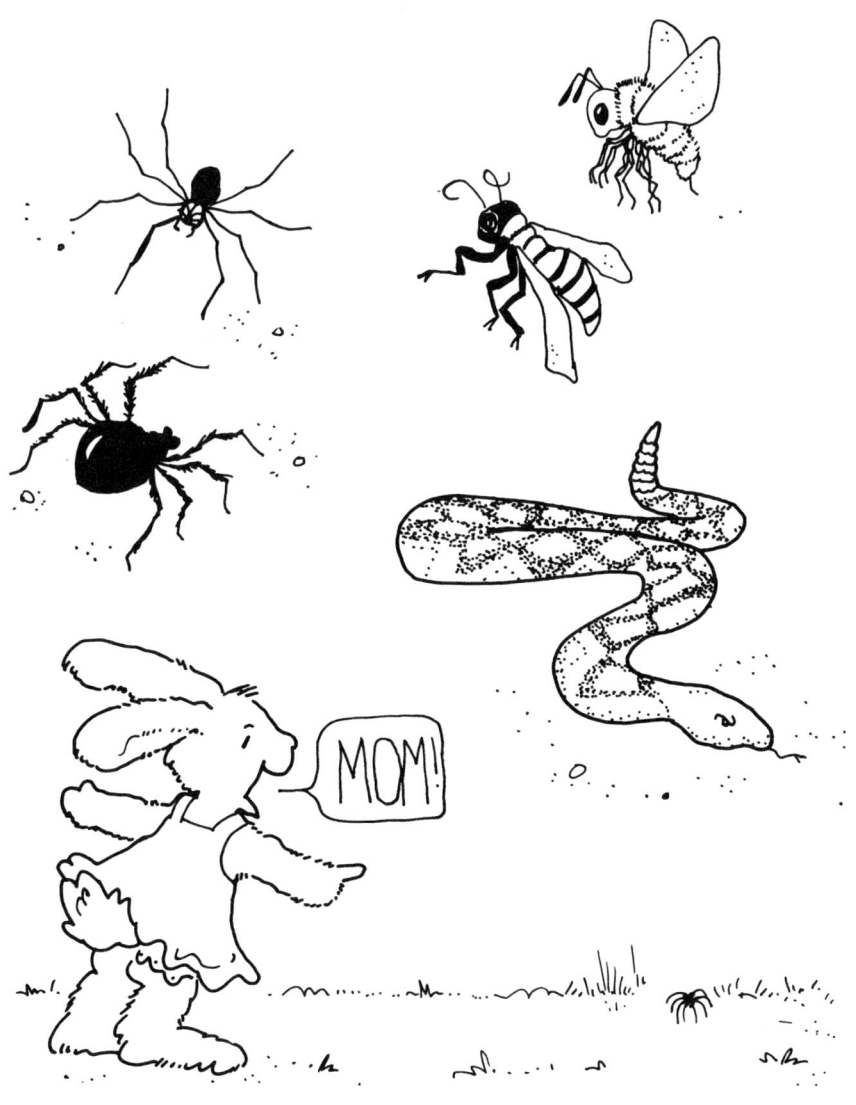

Understanding play safety
©1986 by Incentive Publications. Inc.. Nashville. TN.

Do not put objects
into your eyes,
ears, or nose.
Color the objects
that should not
be put into your
nose, ears or
eyes.

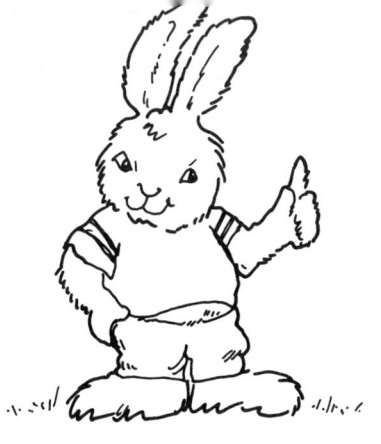

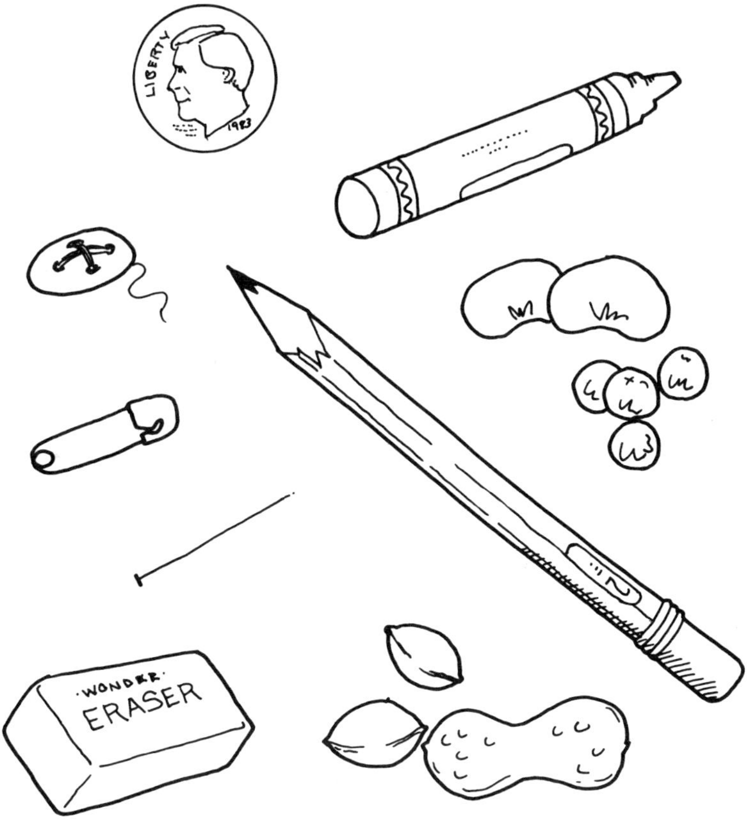

Always wear your shoes when you play
  outside.
There may be sharp sticks, stones or
  broken glass around.
Circle three things that could hurt
  Tonya's feet.

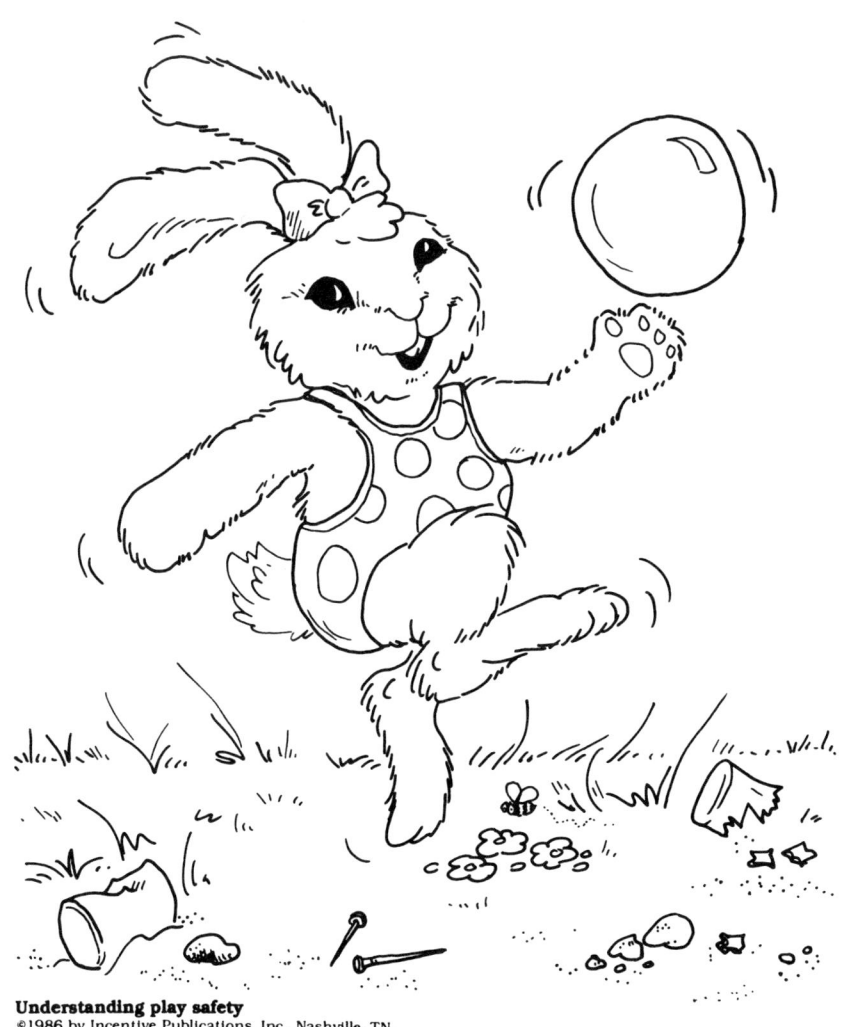

Understanding play safety
©1986 by Incentive Publications, Inc., Nashville, TN.

Check the safety rules below that you always follow.

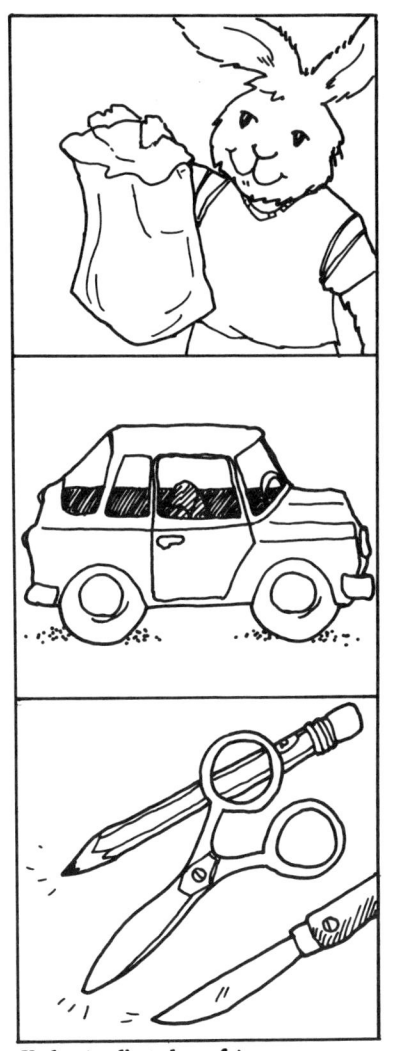

Never put plastic bags over your head.

Never get into an empty automobile.

Always point sharp objects down and never run with them.

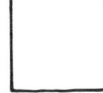

Never play with fire.
You might get burned!
Write this rule.

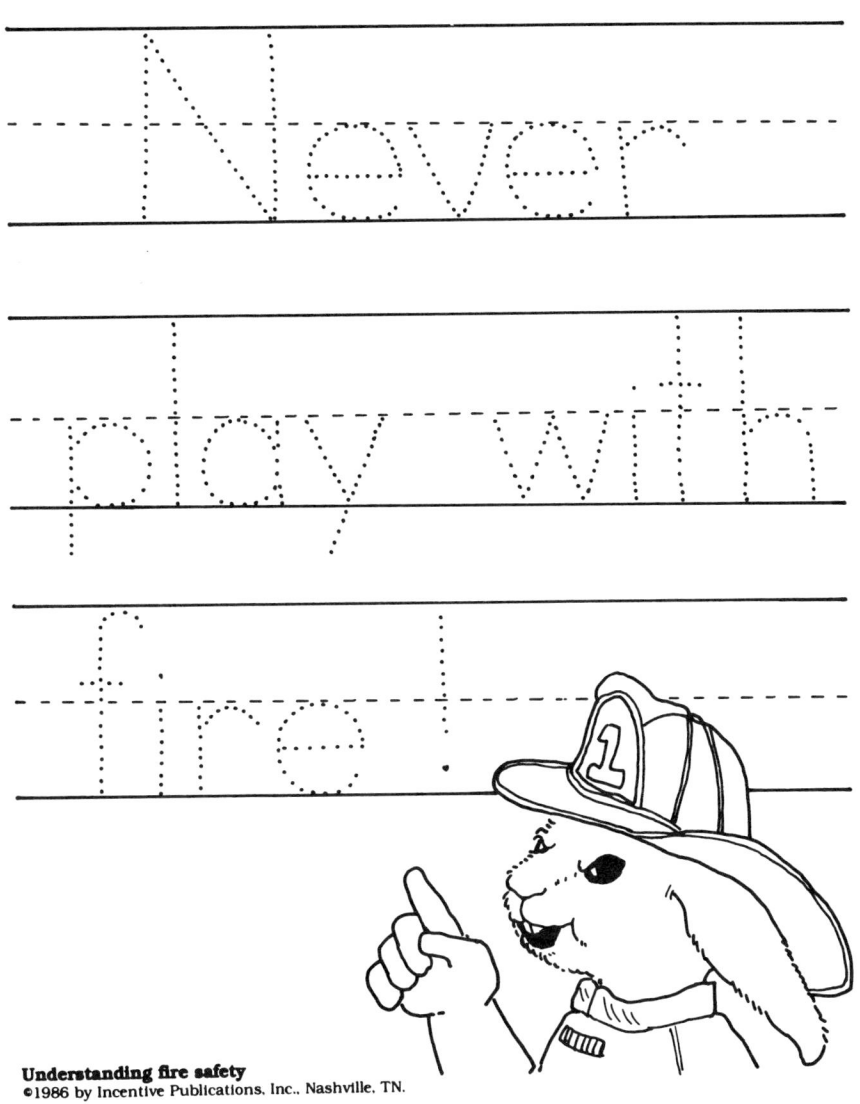

If there is a fire or smoke in your house, get out and call the fire department.
Color this fire hat red.
Write the phone number of your fire department below.

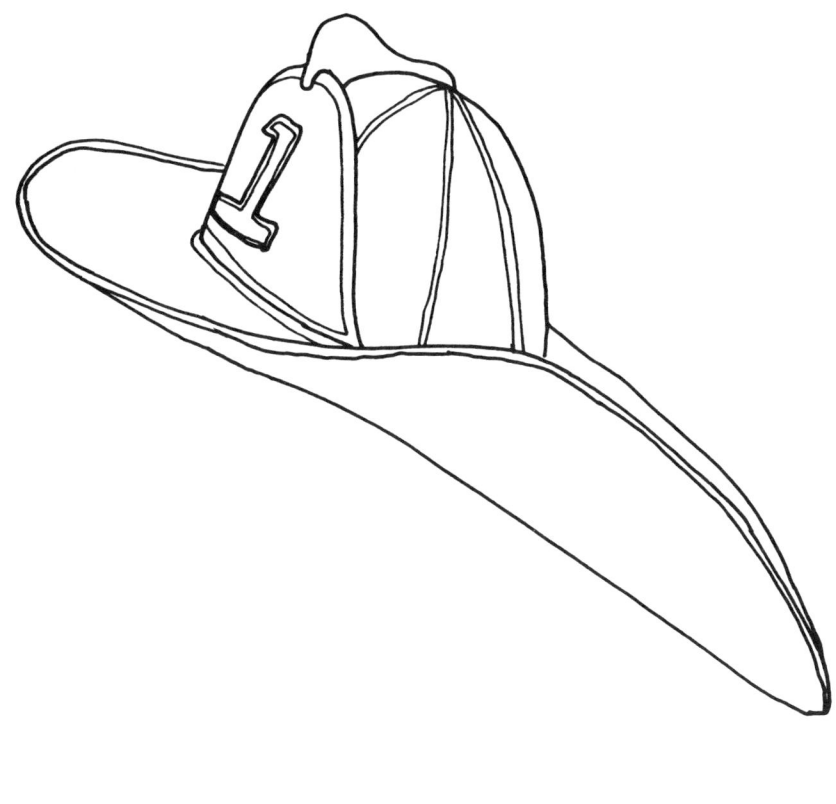

©1986 by Incentive Publications, Inc., Nashville, TN.

If your clothes catch on fire, do you
know what you should do?
Trace the words and color the pictures
to find out.

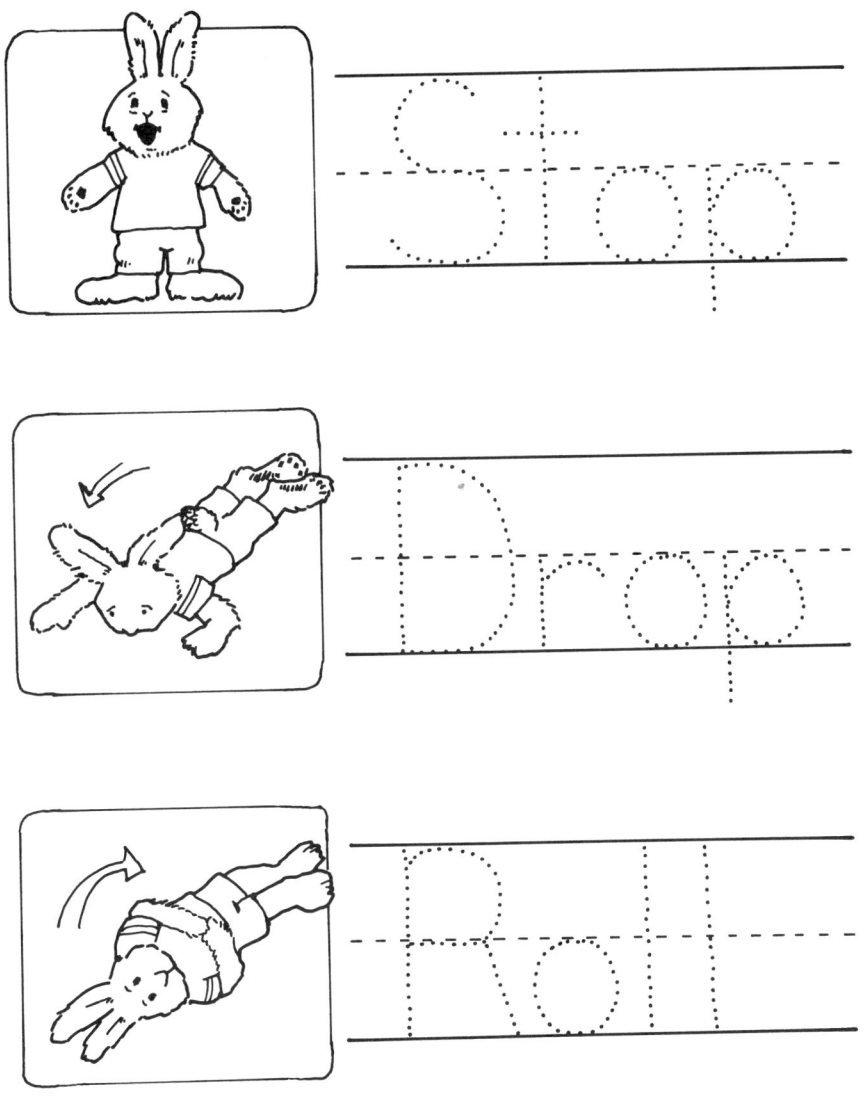

Smoke can make people very sick.
If you wake up and your room is full of
  smoke, crawl along the floor to the
  nearest exit.
Help Tony find the nearest exit.

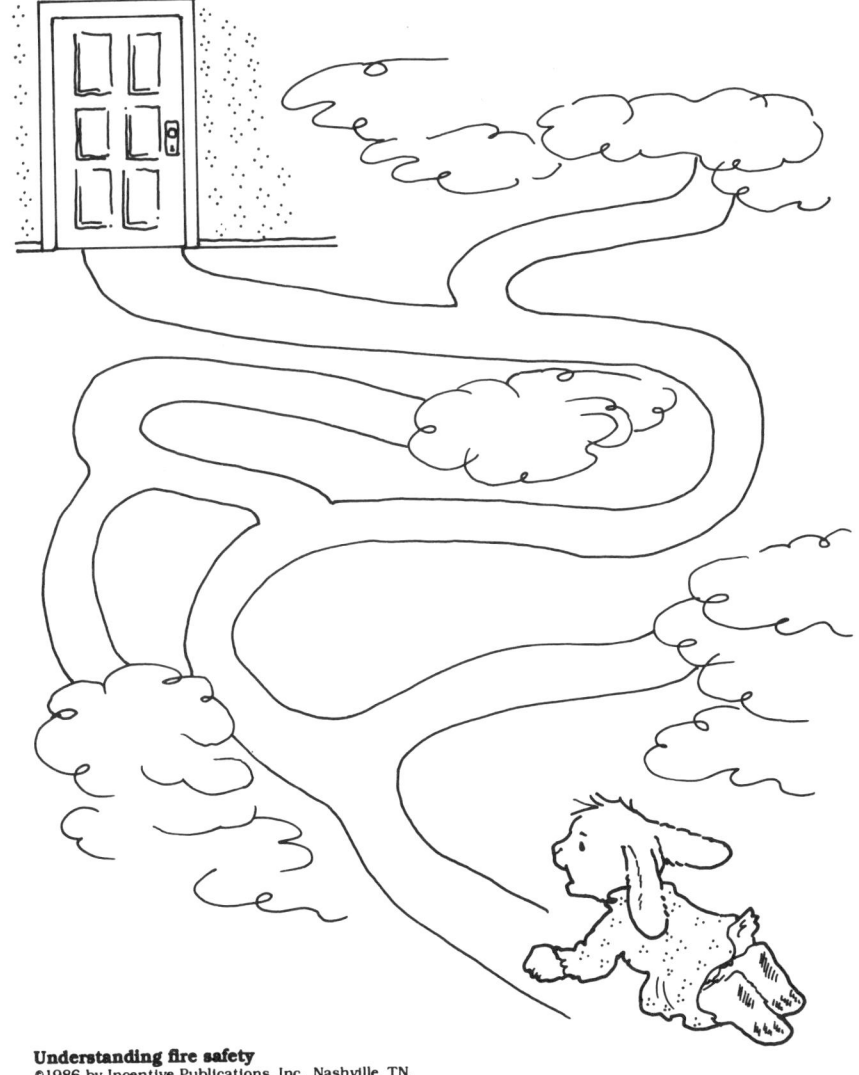

Understanding fire safety
©1986 by Incentive Publications. Inc., Nashville. TN.

Signs help us communicate.
Color each sign and say what it means.

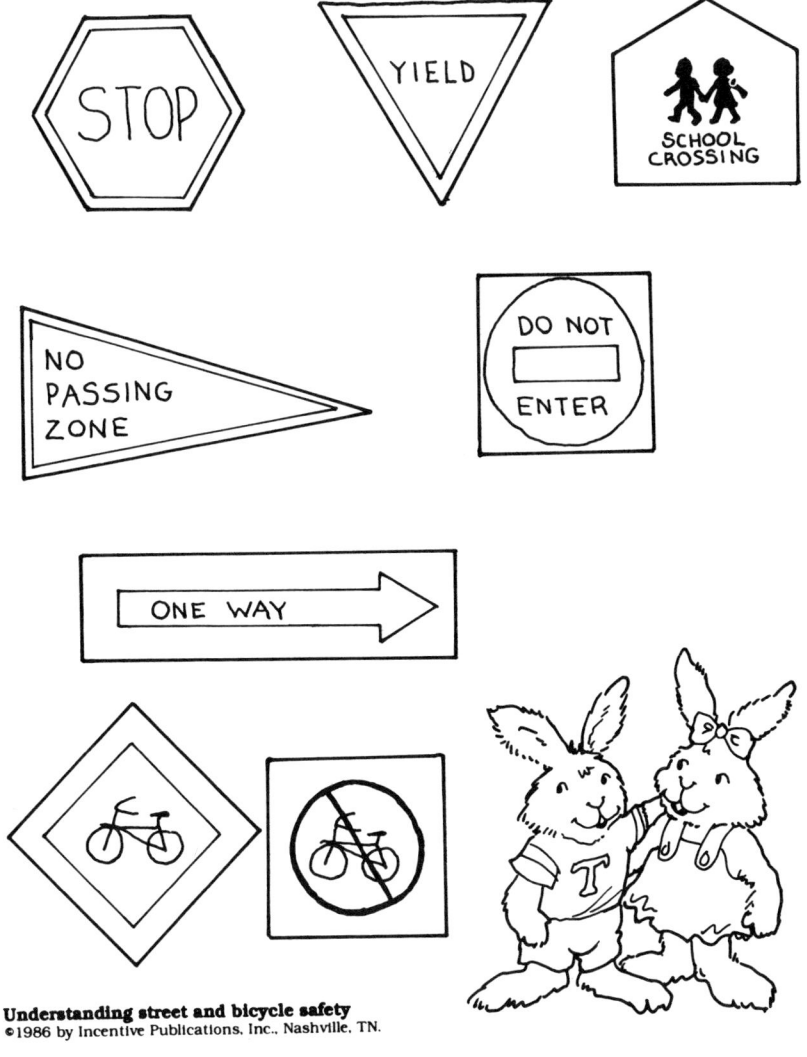

Understanding street and bicycle safety
© 1986 by Incentive Publications, Inc., Nashville, TN.

This traffic light uses colors to tell people when to stop and go. Color the circles and say what they mean.

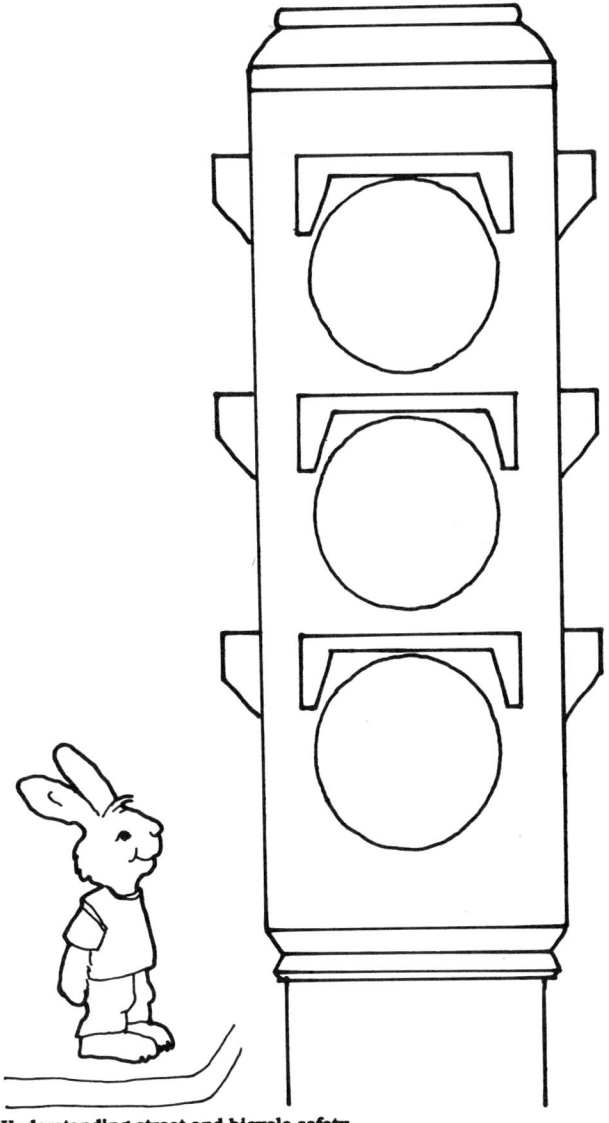

Understanding street and bicycle safety
©1986 by Incentive Publications, Inc., Nashville, TN.

Use hand signals when riding your bike to tell others what you intend to do.
Practice making the signals below.

This is the signal for turning left.

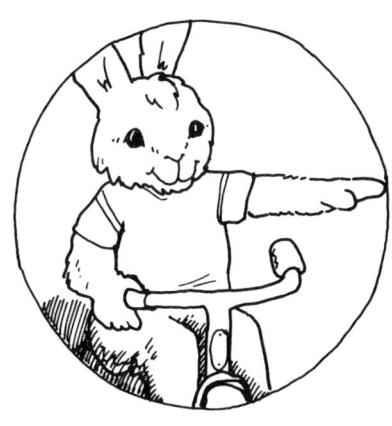

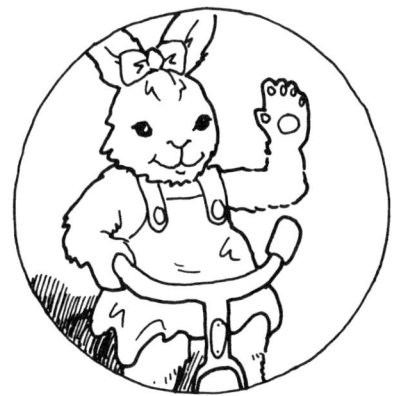

This is the signal for turning right.

This is the signal for stopping.

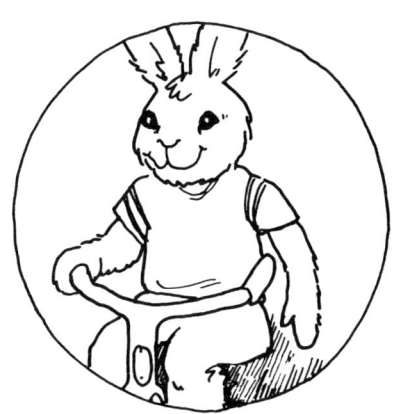

Understanding street and bicycle safety
©1986 by Incentive Publications, Inc., Nashville, TN.

When riding your bike:
- Ride on the right side of the road.
- Obey traffic signs.
- Don't carry riders.

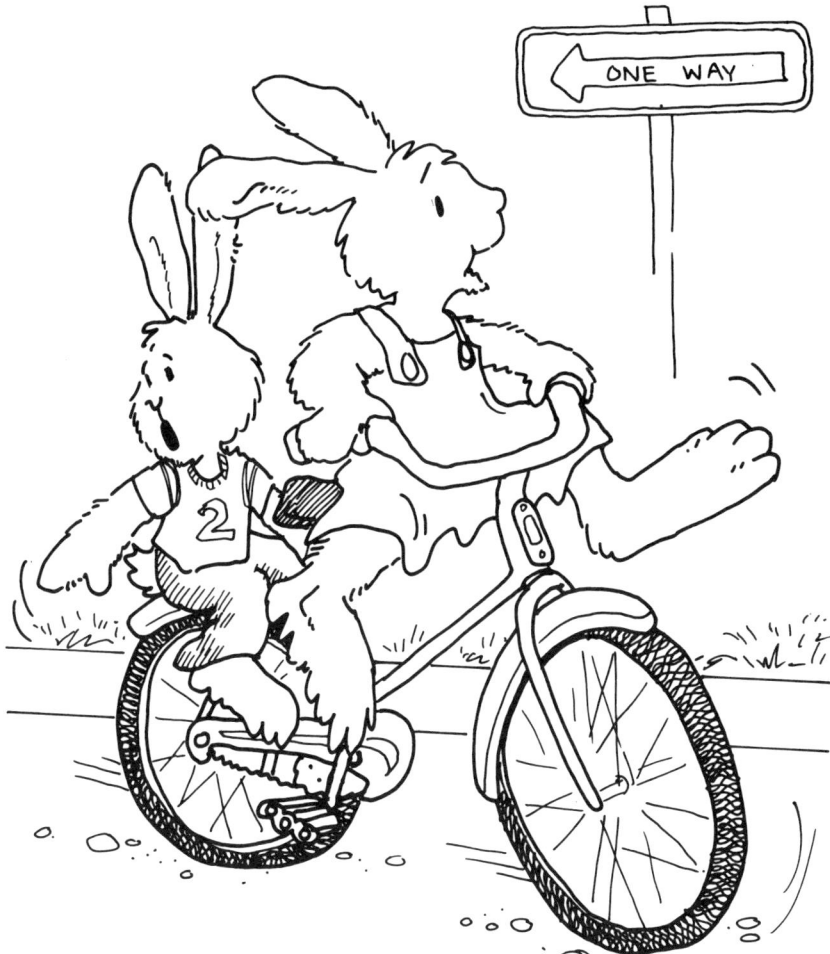

Color the picture and circle the rules which Tony and Tonya are not obeying.

Understanding street and bicycle safety
©1986 by Incentive Publications, Inc., Nashville, TN.

In rainy weather, wear light or brightly colored clothing so others can see you.
Color this raincoat a color that could be seen if it were dark and rainy.

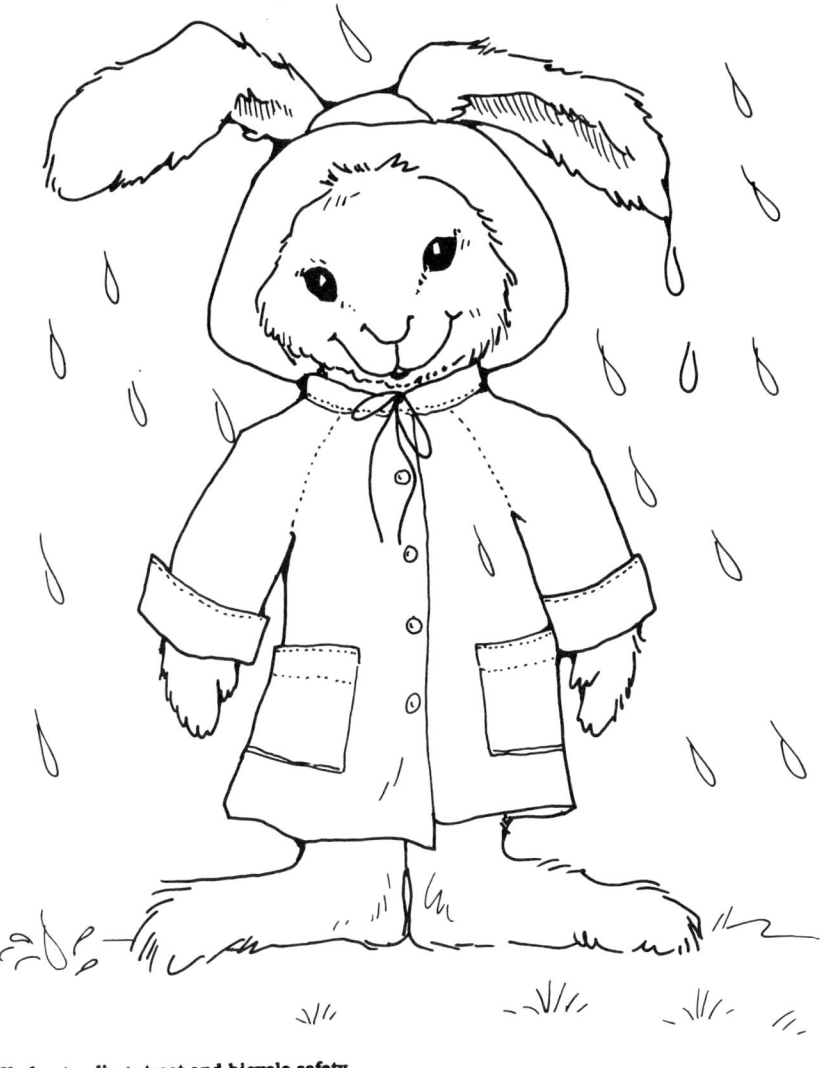

Understanding street and bicycle safety
©1986 by Incentive Publications. Inc.. Nashville. TN.

Check the safety rules below that you always follow.

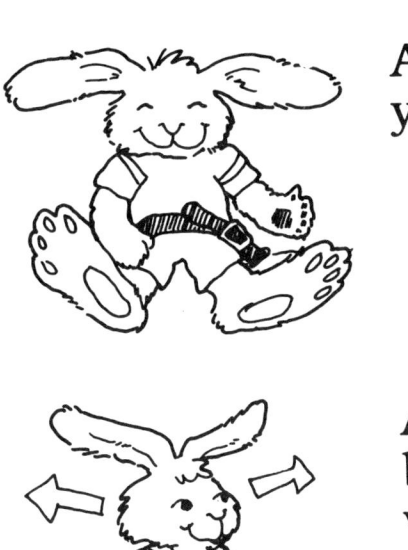 Always wear
your seatbelt.

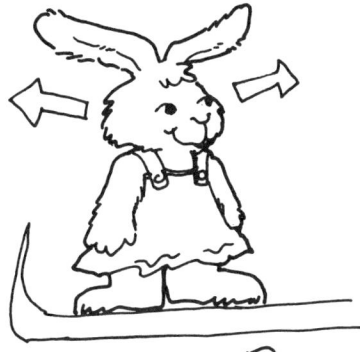 Always look
both ways
when crossing
the street.

 Always walk
your bicycle
across a busy
intersection.

Understanding street and bicycle safety
©1986 by Incentive Publications, Inc., Nashville, TN.

_____

is a

SAFETY SPECIALIST

and knows these important rules:

☐ I know my full name, address and phone number.

☐ I never get in a car or leave with anyone I don't know.

☐ I never accept treats from strangers.

☐ I never wander away from the group when I am playing outside.

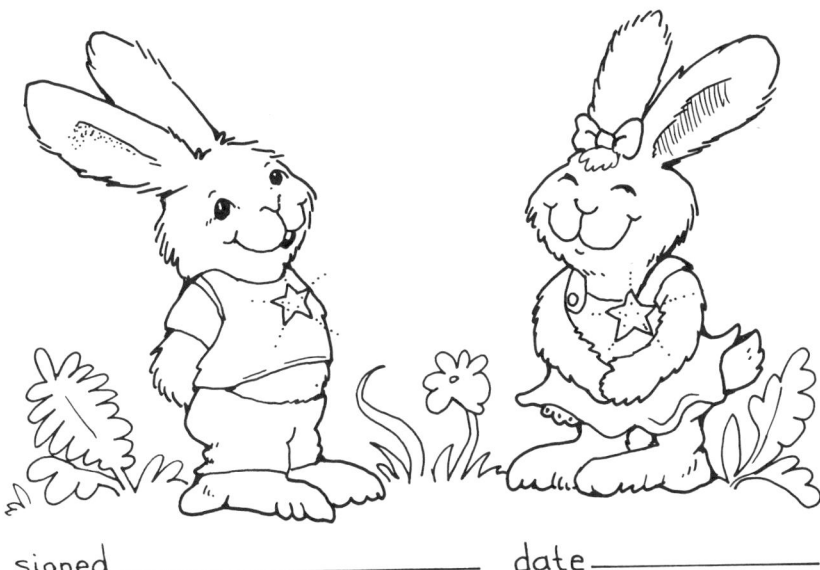

signed _____ date_____

EVERYDAY ACTIVITIES AND PROJECTS FOR CHILDREN
Ready to Learn About Safety

- Help your child make road signs and traffic lights out of construction paper, paint, sticks or other art supplies.

- Encourage your child to use the signs in ordinary, everyday play both outside and in, so that he will become familiar with them. This is also a good way to teach beginning reading skills.

- Encourage a familiarity with and understanding of community helpers by visiting the local fire station, police station and other places where people who "help" work.

- Teach your child about basic differences in plants and animals by taking walks around the neighborhood, visiting zoos and pet shops, reading books and poems and looking at pictures.

- Help your child make a list of "safety rules" to put up in her room. This serves as a concrete reminder of safe ways to act.

- Tell stories, both old favorites and new ones. Point out safety rules in each story. Ask meaningful questions about consequences of rules not followed, etc.